This Log Book Belongs To:

_____

_____

Copyright © 2019 Ellejoy Journals
www.ellejoy.net
All rights reserved.

Receive a free gift

when you subscribe to our mailing list at

www.ellejoy.net

Blood Sugar Log

	BEFORE	AFTER	INSULIN	NOTES
breakfast				
lunch				
dinner				
snack				
bedtime				

· ·

Activity Log

water: ☐☐☐☐☐☐☐

feeling: _____

ACTIVITY TYPE	REPS/DURATION	INTENSITY	CALORIES BURNED

· ·

Notes

_____
_____
_____
_____
_____
_____
_____
_____
_____
_____
_____
_____

Food Log

	FOOD ITEM	CALORIES	CARBS	SUGARS	FIBER	PROTEIN
BREAKFAST						
	TOTAL					
LUNCH						
	TOTAL					
DINNER						
	TOTAL					
SNACKS						
	TOTAL					
SUM	TOTAL FOR THE DAY					

Blood Sugar Log

	BEFORE	AFTER	INSULIN	NOTES
breakfast				
lunch				
dinner				
snack				
bedtime				

Activity Log

water: ▯▯▯▯▯▯▯

feeling: _____

ACTIVITY TYPE	REPS/DURATION	INTENSITY	CALORIES BURNED

Notes

_____
_____
_____
_____
_____
_____
_____
_____
_____

Food Log

	FOOD ITEM	CALORIES	CARBS	SUGARS	FIBER	PROTEIN
BREAKFAST						
	TOTAL					
LUNCH						
	TOTAL					
DINNER						
	TOTAL					
SNACKS						
	TOTAL					
SUM	TOTAL FOR THE DAY					

Blood Sugar Log

	BEFORE	AFTER	INSULIN	NOTES
breakfast				
lunch				
dinner				
snack				
bedtime				

Activity Log

water: ☐☐☐☐☐☐☐

feeling: _____

ACTIVITY TYPE	REPS/DURATION	INTENSITY	CALORIES BURNED

Notes

_____
_____
_____
_____
_____
_____
_____
_____

Food Log

	FOOD ITEM	CALORIES	CARBS	SUGARS	FIBER	PROTEIN
BREAKFAST						
	TOTAL					
LUNCH						
	TOTAL					
DINNER						
	TOTAL					
SNACKS						
	TOTAL					
SUM	TOTAL FOR THE DAY					

Blood Sugar Log

	BEFORE	AFTER	INSULIN	NOTES
breakfast				
lunch				
dinner				
snack				
bedtime				

••

Activity Log

water: ☐☐☐☐☐☐☐   feeling: _____

ACTIVITY TYPE	REPS/DURATION	INTENSITY	CALORIES BURNED

••

Notes

_____
_____
_____
_____
_____
_____
_____
_____
_____
_____

Food Log

	FOOD ITEM	CALORIES	CARBS	SUGARS	FIBER	PROTEIN
BREAKFAST						
	TOTAL					
LUNCH						
	TOTAL					
DINNER						
	TOTAL					
SNACKS						
	TOTAL					
SUM	TOTAL FOR THE DAY					

Blood Sugar Log

	BEFORE	AFTER	INSULIN	NOTES
breakfast				
lunch				
dinner				
snack				
bedtime				

• •

Activity Log

water: ▯▯▯▯▯▯▯

feeling: _____

ACTIVITY TYPE	REPS/DURATION	INTENSITY	CALORIES BURNED

• •

Notes

_____
_____
_____
_____
_____
_____
_____
_____
_____
_____

Food Log

	FOOD ITEM	CALORIES	CARBS	SUGARS	FIBER	PROTEIN
BREAKFAST						
	TOTAL					
LUNCH						
	TOTAL					
DINNER						
	TOTAL					
SNACKS						
	TOTAL					
SUM	TOTAL FOR THE DAY					

Blood Sugar Log

	BEFORE	AFTER	INSULIN	NOTES
breakfast				
lunch				
dinner				
snack				
bedtime				

Activity Log

water: ☐☐☐☐☐☐☐

feeling: _____

ACTIVITY TYPE	REPS/DURATION	INTENSITY	CALORIES BURNED

Notes

_____
_____
_____
_____
_____
_____
_____
_____
_____

Food Log

	FOOD ITEM	CALORIES	CARBS	SUGARS	FIBER	PROTEIN
BREAKFAST						
	TOTAL					
LUNCH						
	TOTAL					
DINNER						
	TOTAL					
SNACKS						
	TOTAL					
SUM	TOTAL FOR THE DAY					

Blood Sugar Log

	BEFORE	AFTER	INSULIN	NOTES
breakfast				
lunch				
dinner				
snack				
bedtime				

Activity Log

water:

feeling:

ACTIVITY TYPE	REPS/DURATION	INTENSITY	CALORIES BURNED

Notes

Food Log

	FOOD ITEM	CALORIES	CARBS	SUGARS	FIBER	PROTEIN
BREAKFAST						
	TOTAL					
LUNCH						
	TOTAL					
DINNER						
	TOTAL					
SNACKS						
	TOTAL					
SUM	TOTAL FOR THE DAY					

Blood Sugar Log

	BEFORE	AFTER	INSULIN	NOTES
breakfast				
lunch				
dinner				
snack				
bedtime				

Activity Log

water: ☐☐☐☐☐☐☐

feeling: _____

ACTIVITY TYPE	REPS/DURATION	INTENSITY	CALORIES BURNED

Notes

_____
_____
_____
_____
_____
_____
_____
_____
_____
_____

Food Log

	FOOD ITEM	CALORIES	CARBS	SUGARS	FIBER	PROTEIN
BREAKFAST						
	TOTAL					
LUNCH						
	TOTAL					
DINNER						
	TOTAL					
SNACKS						
	TOTAL					
SUM	TOTAL FOR THE DAY					

Blood Sugar Log

	BEFORE	AFTER	INSULIN	NOTES
breakfast				
lunch				
dinner				
snack				
bedtime				

Activity Log

water: ☐☐☐☐☐☐☐

feeling: _____

ACTIVITY TYPE	REPS/DURATION	INTENSITY	CALORIES BURNED

Notes

_____
_____
_____
_____
_____
_____
_____
_____
_____
_____

Food Log

	FOOD ITEM	CALORIES	CARBS	SUGARS	FIBER	PROTEIN
BREAKFAST						
	TOTAL					
LUNCH						
	TOTAL					
DINNER						
	TOTAL					
SNACKS						
	TOTAL					
SUM	TOTAL FOR THE DAY					

Blood Sugar Log

	BEFORE	AFTER	INSULIN	NOTES
breakfast				
lunch				
dinner				
snack				
bedtime				

•••

Activity Log

water: ☐☐☐☐☐☐☐

feeling: _____

ACTIVITY TYPE	REPS/DURATION	INTENSITY	CALORIES BURNED

•••

Notes

_____
_____
_____
_____
_____
_____
_____
_____
_____
_____

Food Log

	FOOD ITEM	CALORIES	CARBS	SUGARS	FIBER	PROTEIN
BREAKFAST						
	TOTAL					
LUNCH						
	TOTAL					
DINNER						
	TOTAL					
SNACKS						
	TOTAL					
SUM	TOTAL FOR THE DAY					

Blood Sugar Log

	BEFORE	AFTER	INSULIN	NOTES
breakfast				
lunch				
dinner				
snack				
bedtime				

Activity Log

water: ☐☐☐☐☐☐☐

feeling: _____

ACTIVITY TYPE	REPS/DURATION	INTENSITY	CALORIES BURNED

Notes

_____
_____
_____
_____
_____
_____
_____
_____
_____

Food Log

	FOOD ITEM	CALORIES	CARBS	SUGARS	FIBER	PROTEIN
BREAKFAST						
	TOTAL					
LUNCH						
	TOTAL					
DINNER						
	TOTAL					
SNACKS						
	TOTAL					
SUM	TOTAL FOR THE DAY					

Blood Sugar Log

	BEFORE	AFTER	INSULIN	NOTES
breakfast				
lunch				
dinner				
snack				
bedtime				

• •

Activity Log

water: ☐☐☐☐☐☐☐   feeling: _____

ACTIVITY TYPE	REPS/DURATION	INTENSITY	CALORIES BURNED

• •

Notes

_____
_____
_____
_____
_____
_____
_____
_____
_____
_____

Food Log

	FOOD ITEM	CALORIES	CARBS	SUGARS	FIBER	PROTEIN
BREAKFAST						
	TOTAL					
LUNCH						
	TOTAL					
DINNER						
	TOTAL					
SNACKS						
	TOTAL					
SUM	TOTAL FOR THE DAY					

Blood Sugar Log

	BEFORE	AFTER	INSULIN	NOTES
breakfast				
lunch				
dinner				
snack				
bedtime				

··

Activity Log

water: ☐☐☐☐☐☐☐☐   feeling: _____

ACTIVITY TYPE	REPS/DURATION	INTENSITY	CALORIES BURNED

··

Notes

_____
_____
_____
_____
_____
_____
_____
_____
_____

Food Log

	FOOD ITEM	CALORIES	CARBS	SUGARS	FIBER	PROTEIN
BREAKFAST						
	TOTAL					
LUNCH						
	TOTAL					
DINNER						
	TOTAL					
SNACKS						
	TOTAL					
SUM	TOTAL FOR THE DAY					

Blood Sugar Log

	BEFORE	AFTER	INSULIN	NOTES
breakfast				
lunch				
dinner				
snack				
bedtime				

Activity Log

water: ☐☐☐☐☐☐☐

feeling: _____

ACTIVITY TYPE	REPS/DURATION	INTENSITY	CALORIES BURNED

Notes

_____
_____
_____
_____
_____
_____
_____
_____
_____

Food Log

	FOOD ITEM	CALORIES	CARBS	SUGARS	FIBER	PROTEIN
BREAKFAST						
	TOTAL					
LUNCH						
	TOTAL					
DINNER						
	TOTAL					
SNACKS						
	TOTAL					
SUM	TOTAL FOR THE DAY					

Blood Sugar Log

	BEFORE	AFTER	INSULIN	NOTES
breakfast				
lunch				
dinner				
snack				
bedtime				

Activity Log

water: ▯▯▯▯▯▯▯

feeling: _____

ACTIVITY TYPE	REPS/DURATION	INTENSITY	CALORIES BURNED

Notes

_____
_____
_____
_____
_____
_____
_____
_____
_____

Food Log

	FOOD ITEM	CALORIES	CARBS	SUGARS	FIBER	PROTEIN
BREAKFAST						
	TOTAL					
LUNCH						
	TOTAL					
DINNER						
	TOTAL					
SNACKS						
	TOTAL					
SUM	TOTAL FOR THE DAY					

Blood Sugar Log

	BEFORE	AFTER	INSULIN	NOTES
breakfast				
lunch				
dinner				
snack				
bedtime				

Activity Log

water: ☐☐☐☐☐☐☐

feeling: _____

ACTIVITY TYPE	REPS/DURATION	INTENSITY	CALORIES BURNED

Notes

_____
_____
_____
_____
_____
_____
_____
_____
_____

Food Log

	FOOD ITEM	CALORIES	CARBS	SUGARS	FIBER	PROTEIN
BREAKFAST						
	TOTAL					
LUNCH						
	TOTAL					
DINNER						
	TOTAL					
SNACKS						
	TOTAL					
SUM	TOTAL FOR THE DAY					

Blood Sugar Log

	BEFORE	AFTER	INSULIN	NOTES
breakfast				
lunch				
dinner				
snack				
bedtime				

Activity Log

water:

feeling:

ACTIVITY TYPE	REPS/DURATION	INTENSITY	CALORIES BURNED

Notes

Food Log

	FOOD ITEM	CALORIES	CARBS	SUGARS	FIBER	PROTEIN
BREAKFAST						
	TOTAL					
LUNCH						
	TOTAL					
DINNER						
	TOTAL					
SNACKS						
	TOTAL					
SUM	TOTAL FOR THE DAY					

Blood Sugar Log

	BEFORE	AFTER	INSULIN	NOTES
breakfast				
lunch				
dinner				
snack				
bedtime				

Activity Log

water: ☐☐☐☐☐☐☐

feeling: _____

ACTIVITY TYPE	REPS/DURATION	INTENSITY	CALORIES BURNED

Notes

_____
_____
_____
_____
_____
_____
_____
_____
_____

Food Log

	FOOD ITEM	CALORIES	CARBS	SUGARS	FIBER	PROTEIN
BREAKFAST						
	TOTAL					
LUNCH						
	TOTAL					
DINNER						
	TOTAL					
SNACKS						
	TOTAL					
SUM	TOTAL FOR THE DAY					

Blood Sugar Log

	BEFORE	AFTER	INSULIN	NOTES
breakfast				
lunch				
dinner				
snack				
bedtime				

Activity Log

water: ☐☐☐☐☐☐☐

feeling: _____

ACTIVITY TYPE	REPS/DURATION	INTENSITY	CALORIES BURNED

Notes

_____
_____
_____
_____
_____
_____
_____
_____
_____

Food Log

	FOOD ITEM	CALORIES	CARBS	SUGARS	FIBER	PROTEIN
BREAKFAST						
	TOTAL					
LUNCH						
	TOTAL					
DINNER						
	TOTAL					
SNACKS						
	TOTAL					
SUM	TOTAL FOR THE DAY					

Blood Sugar Log

	BEFORE	AFTER	INSULIN	NOTES
breakfast				
lunch				
dinner				
snack				
bedtime				

Activity Log

water: ☐☐☐☐☐☐☐

feeling: _____

ACTIVITY TYPE	REPS/DURATION	INTENSITY	CALORIES BURNED

Notes

_____
_____
_____
_____
_____
_____
_____
_____
_____

Food Log

	FOOD ITEM	CALORIES	CARBS	SUGARS	FIBER	PROTEIN
BREAKFAST						
	TOTAL					
LUNCH						
	TOTAL					
DINNER						
	TOTAL					
SNACKS						
	TOTAL					
SUM	TOTAL FOR THE DAY					

Blood Sugar Log

	BEFORE	AFTER	INSULIN	NOTES
breakfast				
lunch				
dinner				
snack				
bedtime				

Activity Log

water: ☐☐☐☐☐☐

feeling: _____

ACTIVITY TYPE	REPS/DURATION	INTENSITY	CALORIES BURNED

Notes

_____
_____
_____
_____
_____
_____
_____
_____
_____

Food Log

	FOOD ITEM	CALORIES	CARBS	SUGARS	FIBER	PROTEIN
BREAKFAST						
	TOTAL					
LUNCH						
	TOTAL					
DINNER						
	TOTAL					
SNACKS						
	TOTAL					
SUM	TOTAL FOR THE DAY					

Blood Sugar Log

	BEFORE	AFTER	INSULIN	NOTES
breakfast				
lunch				
dinner				
snack				
bedtime				

••

Activity Log

water: ☐☐☐☐☐☐☐   feeling: _____

ACTIVITY TYPE	REPS/DURATION	INTENSITY	CALORIES BURNED

••

Notes

_____
_____
_____
_____
_____
_____
_____
_____
_____
_____

Food Log

	FOOD ITEM	CALORIES	CARBS	SUGARS	FIBER	PROTEIN
BREAKFAST						
	TOTAL					
LUNCH						
	TOTAL					
DINNER						
	TOTAL					
SNACKS						
	TOTAL					
SUM	TOTAL FOR THE DAY					

Blood Sugar Log

	BEFORE	AFTER	INSULIN	NOTES
breakfast				
lunch				
dinner				
snack				
bedtime				

•••

Activity Log

water:

feeling:

ACTIVITY TYPE	REPS/DURATION	INTENSITY	CALORIES BURNED

•••

Notes

_____
_____
_____
_____
_____
_____
_____
_____
_____
_____

Food Log

	FOOD ITEM	CALORIES	CARBS	SUGARS	FIBER	PROTEIN
BREAKFAST						
	TOTAL					
LUNCH						
	TOTAL					
DINNER						
	TOTAL					
SNACKS						
	TOTAL					
SUM	TOTAL FOR THE DAY					

Blood Sugar Log

	BEFORE	AFTER	INSULIN	NOTES
breakfast				
lunch				
dinner				
snack				
bedtime				

Activity Log

water: ☐☐☐☐☐☐☐

feeling: _____

ACTIVITY TYPE	REPS/DURATION	INTENSITY	CALORIES BURNED

Notes

_____
_____
_____
_____
_____
_____
_____
_____
_____

Food Log

	FOOD ITEM	CALORIES	CARBS	SUGARS	FIBER	PROTEIN
BREAKFAST						
	TOTAL					
LUNCH						
	TOTAL					
DINNER						
	TOTAL					
SNACKS						
	TOTAL					
SUM	TOTAL FOR THE DAY					

Blood Sugar Log

	BEFORE	AFTER	INSULIN	NOTES
breakfast				
lunch				
dinner				
snack				
bedtime				

Activity Log

water:

feeling:

ACTIVITY TYPE	REPS/DURATION	INTENSITY	CALORIES BURNED

Notes

Food Log

	FOOD ITEM	CALORIES	CARBS	SUGARS	FIBER	PROTEIN
BREAKFAST						
	TOTAL					
LUNCH						
	TOTAL					
DINNER						
	TOTAL					
SNACKS						
	TOTAL					
SUM	TOTAL FOR THE DAY					

Blood Sugar Log

	BEFORE	AFTER	INSULIN	NOTES
breakfast				
lunch				
dinner				
snack				
bedtime				

Activity Log

water: ▯▯▯▯▯▯▯

feeling: _____

ACTIVITY TYPE	REPS/DURATION	INTENSITY	CALORIES BURNED

Notes

_____
_____
_____
_____
_____
_____
_____
_____
_____
_____

Food Log

	FOOD ITEM	CALORIES	CARBS	SUGARS	FIBER	PROTEIN
BREAKFAST						
	TOTAL					
LUNCH						
	TOTAL					
DINNER						
	TOTAL					
SNACKS						
	TOTAL					
SUM	TOTAL FOR THE DAY					

Blood Sugar Log

	BEFORE	AFTER	INSULIN	NOTES
breakfast				
lunch				
dinner				
snack				
bedtime				

Activity Log

water: ⬜⬜⬜⬜⬜⬜⬜

feeling: _____

ACTIVITY TYPE	REPS/DURATION	INTENSITY	CALORIES BURNED

Notes

_____
_____
_____
_____
_____
_____
_____
_____
_____

Food Log

	FOOD ITEM	CALORIES	CARBS	SUGARS	FIBER	PROTEIN
BREAKFAST						
	TOTAL					
LUNCH						
	TOTAL					
DINNER						
	TOTAL					
SNACKS						
	TOTAL					
SUM	TOTAL FOR THE DAY					

Blood Sugar Log

	BEFORE	AFTER	INSULIN	NOTES
breakfast				
lunch				
dinner				
snack				
bedtime				

....

Activity Log

water: ☐☐☐☐☐☐☐   feeling: _____

ACTIVITY TYPE	REPS/DURATION	INTENSITY	CALORIES BURNED

....

Notes

_____
_____
_____
_____
_____
_____
_____
_____
_____
_____

Food Log

	FOOD ITEM	CALORIES	CARBS	SUGARS	FIBER	PROTEIN
BREAKFAST						
	TOTAL					
LUNCH						
	TOTAL					
DINNER						
	TOTAL					
SNACKS						
	TOTAL					
SUM	TOTAL FOR THE DAY					

Blood Sugar Log

	BEFORE	AFTER	INSULIN	NOTES
breakfast				
lunch				
dinner				
snack				
bedtime				

• •

Activity Log

water: ☐☐☐☐☐☐☐☐

feeling: _____

ACTIVITY TYPE	REPS/DURATION	INTENSITY	CALORIES BURNED

• •

Notes

_____
_____
_____
_____
_____
_____
_____
_____
_____

Food Log

	FOOD ITEM	CALORIES	CARBS	SUGARS	FIBER	PROTEIN
BREAKFAST						
	TOTAL					
LUNCH						
	TOTAL					
DINNER						
	TOTAL					
SNACKS						
	TOTAL					
SUM	TOTAL FOR THE DAY					

Blood Sugar Log

	BEFORE	AFTER	INSULIN	NOTES
breakfast				
lunch				
dinner				
snack				
bedtime				

• •

Activity Log

water: ☐☐☐☐☐☐☐ feeling: _____

ACTIVITY TYPE	REPS/DURATION	INTENSITY	CALORIES BURNED

• •

Notes

_____
_____
_____
_____
_____
_____
_____
_____
_____
_____

Food Log

	FOOD ITEM	CALORIES	CARBS	SUGARS	FIBER	PROTEIN
BREAKFAST						
	TOTAL					
LUNCH						
	TOTAL					
DINNER						
	TOTAL					
SNACKS						
	TOTAL					
SUM	TOTAL FOR THE DAY					

Blood Sugar Log

	BEFORE	AFTER	INSULIN	NOTES
breakfast				
lunch				
dinner				
snack				
bedtime				

•••

Activity Log

water: ☐☐☐☐☐☐☐☐

feeling: _____

ACTIVITY TYPE	REPS/DURATION	INTENSITY	CALORIES BURNED

•••

Notes

_____
_____
_____
_____
_____
_____
_____
_____
_____
_____

Food Log

	FOOD ITEM	CALORIES	CARBS	SUGARS	FIBER	PROTEIN
BREAKFAST						
	TOTAL					
LUNCH						
	TOTAL					
DINNER						
	TOTAL					
SNACKS						
	TOTAL					
SUM	TOTAL FOR THE DAY					

Blood Sugar Log

	BEFORE	AFTER	INSULIN	NOTES
breakfast				
lunch				
dinner				
snack				
bedtime				

Activity Log

water: ▢▢▢▢▢▢▢

feeling: _____

ACTIVITY TYPE	REPS/DURATION	INTENSITY	CALORIES BURNED

Notes

_____
_____
_____
_____
_____
_____
_____
_____
_____

Food Log

	FOOD ITEM	CALORIES	CARBS	SUGARS	FIBER	PROTEIN
BREAKFAST						
	TOTAL					
LUNCH						
	TOTAL					
DINNER						
	TOTAL					
SNACKS						
	TOTAL					
SUM	TOTAL FOR THE DAY					

Blood Sugar Log

	BEFORE	AFTER	INSULIN	NOTES
breakfast				
lunch				
dinner				
snack				
bedtime				

Activity Log

water: ▢▢▢▢▢▢▢

feeling: _____

ACTIVITY TYPE	REPS/DURATION	INTENSITY	CALORIES BURNED

Notes

_____
_____
_____
_____
_____
_____
_____
_____
_____

Food Log

	FOOD ITEM	CALORIES	CARBS	SUGARS	FIBER	PROTEIN
BREAKFAST						
	TOTAL					
LUNCH						
	TOTAL					
DINNER						
	TOTAL					
SNACKS						
	TOTAL					
SUM	TOTAL FOR THE DAY					

Blood Sugar Log

	BEFORE	AFTER	INSULIN	NOTES
breakfast				
lunch				
dinner				
snack				
bedtime				

Activity Log

water: ☐☐☐☐☐☐☐

feeling: _____

ACTIVITY TYPE	REPS/DURATION	INTENSITY	CALORIES BURNED

Notes

_____
_____
_____
_____
_____
_____
_____
_____
_____
_____

Food Log

	FOOD ITEM	CALORIES	CARBS	SUGARS	FIBER	PROTEIN
BREAKFAST						
	TOTAL					
LUNCH						
	TOTAL					
DINNER						
	TOTAL					
SNACKS						
	TOTAL					
SUM	TOTAL FOR THE DAY					

Blood Sugar Log

	BEFORE	AFTER	INSULIN	NOTES
breakfast				
lunch				
dinner				
snack				
bedtime				

••

Activity Log

water: ☐☐☐☐☐☐☐   feeling: _____

ACTIVITY TYPE	REPS/DURATION	INTENSITY	CALORIES BURNED

••

Notes

_____
_____
_____
_____
_____
_____
_____
_____
_____

Food Log

	FOOD ITEM	CALORIES	CARBS	SUGARS	FIBER	PROTEIN
BREAKFAST						
	TOTAL					
LUNCH						
	TOTAL					
DINNER						
	TOTAL					
SNACKS						
	TOTAL					
SUM	TOTAL FOR THE DAY					

Blood Sugar Log

	BEFORE	AFTER	INSULIN	NOTES
breakfast				
lunch				
dinner				
snack				
bedtime				

• •

Activity Log

water: ▯▯▯▯▯▯▯

feeling: _____

ACTIVITY TYPE	REPS/DURATION	INTENSITY	CALORIES BURNED

• •

Notes

_____
_____
_____
_____
_____
_____
_____
_____
_____

Food Log

	FOOD ITEM	CALORIES	CARBS	SUGARS	FIBER	PROTEIN
BREAKFAST						
	TOTAL					
LUNCH						
	TOTAL					
DINNER						
	TOTAL					
SNACKS						
	TOTAL					
SUM	TOTAL FOR THE DAY					

Blood Sugar Log

	BEFORE	AFTER	INSULIN	NOTES
breakfast				
lunch				
dinner				
snack				
bedtime				

•••

Activity Log

water:
☐☐☐☐☐☐

feeling: _____

ACTIVITY TYPE	REPS/DURATION	INTENSITY	CALORIES BURNED

•••

Notes

_____
_____
_____
_____
_____
_____
_____
_____
_____
_____

Food Log

	FOOD ITEM	CALORIES	CARBS	SUGARS	FIBER	PROTEIN
BREAKFAST						
	TOTAL					
LUNCH						
	TOTAL					
DINNER						
	TOTAL					
SNACKS						
	TOTAL					
SUM	TOTAL FOR THE DAY					

Blood Sugar Log

	BEFORE	AFTER	INSULIN	NOTES
breakfast				
lunch				
dinner				
snack				
bedtime				

Activity Log

water: ▯▯▯▯▯▯▯

feeling: _____

ACTIVITY TYPE	REPS/DURATION	INTENSITY	CALORIES BURNED

Notes

_____
_____
_____
_____
_____
_____
_____
_____
_____

Food Log

	FOOD ITEM	CALORIES	CARBS	SUGARS	FIBER	PROTEIN
BREAKFAST						
	TOTAL					
LUNCH						
	TOTAL					
DINNER						
	TOTAL					
SNACKS						
	TOTAL					
SUM	TOTAL FOR THE DAY					

Blood Sugar Log

	BEFORE	AFTER	INSULIN	NOTES
breakfast				
lunch				
dinner				
snack				
bedtime				

• •

Activity Log

water: ▯▯▯▯▯▯▯   feeling: _____

ACTIVITY TYPE	REPS/DURATION	INTENSITY	CALORIES BURNED

• •

Notes

_____
_____
_____
_____
_____
_____
_____
_____
_____

Food Log

	FOOD ITEM	CALORIES	CARBS	SUGARS	FIBER	PROTEIN
BREAKFAST						
	TOTAL					
LUNCH						
	TOTAL					
DINNER						
	TOTAL					
SNACKS						
	TOTAL					
SUM	TOTAL FOR THE DAY					

Blood Sugar Log

	BEFORE	AFTER	INSULIN	NOTES
breakfast				
lunch				
dinner				
snack				
bedtime				

Activity Log

water: ⬜⬜⬜⬜⬜⬜⬜

feeling: _____

ACTIVITY TYPE	REPS/DURATION	INTENSITY	CALORIES BURNED

Notes

_____
_____
_____
_____
_____
_____
_____
_____
_____
_____

Food Log

	FOOD ITEM	CALORIES	CARBS	SUGARS	FIBER	PROTEIN
BREAKFAST						
	TOTAL					
LUNCH						
	TOTAL					
DINNER						
	TOTAL					
SNACKS						
	TOTAL					
SUM	TOTAL FOR THE DAY					

Blood Sugar Log

	BEFORE	AFTER	INSULIN	NOTES
breakfast				
lunch				
dinner				
snack				
bedtime				

• •

Activity Log

water: ▢▢▢▢▢▢▢

feeling: _____

ACTIVITY TYPE	REPS/DURATION	INTENSITY	CALORIES BURNED

• •

Notes

_____
_____
_____
_____
_____
_____
_____
_____
_____

Food Log

	FOOD ITEM	CALORIES	CARBS	SUGARS	FIBER	PROTEIN
BREAKFAST						
	TOTAL					
LUNCH						
	TOTAL					
DINNER						
	TOTAL					
SNACKS						
	TOTAL					
SUM	TOTAL FOR THE DAY					

Blood Sugar Log

	BEFORE	AFTER	INSULIN	NOTES
breakfast				
lunch				
dinner				
snack				
bedtime				

Activity Log

water: ☐☐☐☐☐☐☐

feeling: _____

ACTIVITY TYPE	REPS/DURATION	INTENSITY	CALORIES BURNED

Notes

_____
_____
_____
_____
_____
_____
_____
_____

Food Log

	FOOD ITEM	CALORIES	CARBS	SUGARS	FIBER	PROTEIN
BREAKFAST						
	TOTAL					
LUNCH						
	TOTAL					
DINNER						
	TOTAL					
SNACKS						
	TOTAL					
SUM	TOTAL FOR THE DAY					

Blood Sugar Log

	BEFORE	AFTER	INSULIN	NOTES
breakfast				
lunch				
dinner				
snack				
bedtime				

••

Activity Log

water: ☐☐☐☐☐☐☐   feeling: _____

ACTIVITY TYPE	REPS/DURATION	INTENSITY	CALORIES BURNED

••

Notes

_____
_____
_____
_____
_____
_____
_____
_____
_____
_____

Food Log

	FOOD ITEM	CALORIES	CARBS	SUGARS	FIBER	PROTEIN
BREAKFAST						
	TOTAL					
LUNCH						
	TOTAL					
DINNER						
	TOTAL					
SNACKS						
	TOTAL					
SUM	TOTAL FOR THE DAY					

Blood Sugar Log

	BEFORE	AFTER	INSULIN	NOTES
breakfast				
lunch				
dinner				
snack				
bedtime				

Activity Log

water:

feeling:

ACTIVITY TYPE	REPS/DURATION	INTENSITY	CALORIES BURNED

Notes

Food Log

	FOOD ITEM	CALORIES	CARBS	SUGARS	FIBER	PROTEIN
BREAKFAST						
	TOTAL					
LUNCH						
	TOTAL					
DINNER						
	TOTAL					
SNACKS						
	TOTAL					
SUM	TOTAL FOR THE DAY					

Blood Sugar Log

	BEFORE	AFTER	INSULIN	NOTES
breakfast				
lunch				
dinner				
snack				
bedtime				

Activity Log

water: ☐☐☐☐☐☐☐

feeling: _____

ACTIVITY TYPE	REPS/DURATION	INTENSITY	CALORIES BURNED

Notes

_____
_____
_____
_____
_____
_____
_____
_____
_____
_____

Food Log

	FOOD ITEM	CALORIES	CARBS	SUGARS	FIBER	PROTEIN
BREAKFAST						
	TOTAL					
LUNCH						
	TOTAL					
DINNER						
	TOTAL					
SNACKS						
	TOTAL					
SUM	TOTAL FOR THE DAY					

Blood Sugar Log

	BEFORE	AFTER	INSULIN	NOTES
breakfast				
lunch				
dinner				
snack				
bedtime				

•••

Activity Log

water: ☐☐☐☐☐☐☐

feeling: _____

ACTIVITY TYPE	REPS/DURATION	INTENSITY	CALORIES BURNED

•••

Notes

_____
_____
_____
_____
_____
_____
_____
_____
_____
_____

Food Log

	FOOD ITEM	CALORIES	CARBS	SUGARS	FIBER	PROTEIN
BREAKFAST						
	TOTAL					
LUNCH						
	TOTAL					
DINNER						
	TOTAL					
SNACKS						
	TOTAL					
SUM	TOTAL FOR THE DAY					

Blood Sugar Log

	BEFORE	AFTER	INSULIN	NOTES
breakfast				
lunch				
dinner				
snack				
bedtime				

••

Activity Log

water: ⬜⬜⬜⬜⬜⬜⬜

feeling: _____

ACTIVITY TYPE	REPS/DURATION	INTENSITY	CALORIES BURNED

••

Notes

_____
_____
_____
_____
_____
_____
_____
_____
_____

Food Log

	FOOD ITEM	CALORIES	CARBS	SUGARS	FIBER	PROTEIN
BREAKFAST						
	TOTAL					
LUNCH						
	TOTAL					
DINNER						
	TOTAL					
SNACKS						
	TOTAL					
SUM	TOTAL FOR THE DAY					

Blood Sugar Log

	BEFORE	AFTER	INSULIN	NOTES
breakfast				
lunch				
dinner				
snack				
bedtime				

Activity Log

water: ▢▢▢▢▢▢▢

feeling: _____

ACTIVITY TYPE	REPS/DURATION	INTENSITY	CALORIES BURNED

Notes

_____
_____
_____
_____
_____
_____
_____
_____
_____

Food Log

	FOOD ITEM	CALORIES	CARBS	SUGARS	FIBER	PROTEIN
BREAKFAST						
	TOTAL					
LUNCH						
	TOTAL					
DINNER						
	TOTAL					
SNACKS						
	TOTAL					
SUM	TOTAL FOR THE DAY					

Blood Sugar Log

	BEFORE	AFTER	INSULIN	NOTES
breakfast				
lunch				
dinner				
snack				
bedtime				

Activity Log

water:

feeling:

ACTIVITY TYPE	REPS/DURATION	INTENSITY	CALORIES BURNED

Notes

Made in the USA
Las Vegas, NV
26 February 2023

68201684R00059